The A Thru' Z of MR

David Bryant and Simon Blease

Series Editor: Paul R. Goddard

© Clinical Press Ltd. 1997
All rights reserved. No part of this publication may be reproduced, stored in a retrieval system or transmitted in any form or by any means, electronic, mechanical, photocopying, recording or otherwise without the prior permission of the Copyright owner.

Published by:
Clinical Press Limited
Registered Office:
Redland Green Farm
Redland
Bristol, BS6 7HF
UK

Bryant, D. and Blease, S.
The A thru' Z of MR
Medicine: Radiology

ISBN: 1 85457 033 1

An MRI Glossary

Much MRI literature assumes that the reader is conversant with the specialised terms that have developed with the subject. For beginners this is often not the case, and this false assumption may hinder the reader's assimilation of information. The aim of this glossary is to explain these terms in plain language without assuming that the reader has a PhD in physics!

A

● **Adiabatic Fast Passage**
Tissue placed in the magnetic field of a diagnostic MR machine will attain a "bulk magnetic vector". This vector can be rotated by sweeping the frequency of the interrogating radiofrequency wave through the resonant (Larmor) frequencies of the protons in that tissue. The rate of sweep is kept short compared to the relaxation times of these protons and this technique, called adiabatic fast passage is useful in the longer Inversion Recovery sequences. Pulsed adiabatic signals can be used to produce uniform flip angles in compensation for non-uniform radiofrequency fields.

● **Aliasing**
The phenomenon of aliasing is not unique to MR. Therefore an identifying synonym is more often used which is Wraparound. This artifact results from data lying outside the field of view being "wrapped" back into the image. Aliasing occurs in both phase and frequency encoding directions on the final image. Enlarging the field of view can reduce the artifact, but specific measures can be applied to overcome both types of MR aliasing.

Frequency encoded aliasing can be reduced by "oversampling" along this axis. By doubling the rate of data acquisition, which will double the field of view in the frequency encode direction, the effects of aliasing can be removed. The edge of the image can also be attenuated or removed by filtering the higher frequencies from the observed signal.

Phase encoded aliasing data is "wrapped" onto the opposite side of the image. Unfortunately, oversampling doubles the imaging time and so the artifact is usually reduced by either increasing the field of view, altering the phase encoding direction or reducing the sample volume by using a surface coil.

● **Analogue-to-Digital Converter**
The MR signal generated from the tissue under study will be a mass of waveforms known as the free induction decay. To allow for computer storage and manipulation the waveforms must be allocated numerical values or digitized. This occurs in an analogue-to-digital converter (ADC). The signals are samples at microsecond intervals and allocated a numerical value according to their magnitude. The signal may be divided into something like 16384 or 32768 distinct levels. The digitised signal can then be stored prior to processing.

● **Angiography**
Fast imaging sequences can be used to demonstrate flow in vessels. By using subtraction techniques the vessels alone can be imaged.

The technique is still being refined but in its simplest terms it makes use of the phenomenon of "paradoxical enhancement." Also known as Flow Related Enhancement, it refers to the fact that blood flowing into a slice of tissue has only been excited by a single radiofrequency pulse and will retain all its magnetisation. This is referred to as an unsaturated state and is in distinction to the stationary tissue in the slice which will be "partially saturated" or recovering its original magnetisation after the RF pulse. This difference is exploited in order to form the angiogram image. It is important to keep scan times and sequence parameters as short as possible to minimise motion artifact and loss of signal due to blood flowing out of the slice.

There are two main sequence types used to perform MR angiography; Time of Flight (TOF) and Phase Sensitive. The former is more robust and covers larger areas but is prone to signal loss from in-plane flow. The latter is more sensitive to slower flow and it can be adjusted to detect either asterial or venous flow rates (velocity engaging) signal from smaller vessels can be improved by adding Magnetisation Transfer Contrast.

With the development of Ultra-Fast Gradient Echo sequences it is now possible to acquire images in a single breath-hold during the blood pool phase of Gadolinium injection. Although an invasive technique, it allows background detail to be retained.

- **Angular momentum**

Classically the nucleus is imagined as a small planet that is rotating and as such it has angular momentum. Angular momentum is a vector quantity, it has a direction along the axis of the rotation and a magnitude dependent upon the rate of rotation.

- **Anti-parallel**

The spinning properties of nuclei in living tissues will cause them to behave as minute magnets or dipoles. If a strong external magnetic field (called B_0 in MR) is applied, these dipoles can align with (parallel) or against (anti-parallel) the vector of B_0.

The parallel alignment is a lower energy state and so proportionately more nuclei will occupy this condition. The difference is small (in the order of 1 or 2 per million) but it is this excess population in the parallel alignment which contributes to the detectable MR signal since the nuclei in the anti-parallel state will cancel out the signal from the equivalent number of parallel spins. The actual parallel/anti-parallel distribution will be predicted by the Boltzmann equation.

B

- **B_0**

The permanent magnetic field strength of an MR magnet is given the symbol B_0 and is measured in Tesla. For diagnostic MR the usual shorthand for this value is 0.5T, 1.0T, 1.5T etc.

- **B_1**

This is the symbol given to the magnetic field strength of the interrogating radiofrequency wave. B_1 fields are very small in comparison to B_0 and will typically be in the range 5-50µT (10^{-6}T).

- **Binomial Pulse**

This is a technique used to suppress the signal from water protons in MR spectroscopy. It is comprised of a train of two or more radiofrequency pulses as in 11, 12, 1331 etc respectively. Although each individual pulse is broadband, the final excitation spectrum of the composite pulse is limited. The binomial pulse has widespread use in the acquisition of ^1H spectra where the large signals from water and lipid can be attenuated by carefully positioning the excitation profile over the spectrum.

- **BOLD**

A functional MRI mechanism which is Blood Oxygen Level Dependent. Deoxyhaemoglobin is paramagnetic. As a tissue utilises oxygen, the proportion of this molecule will rise which produces a visible alteration in the MR signal. The main effect is a local dephasing which will cause a reduction in $T_2\star$. However, blood supply will increase with increasing oxygen utilisation which will reduce the proportion of Deoxyhaemoglobin and result in an increase in signal.

● **Boltzmann Distribution**
Nuclei in thermal equilibrium can exist in high or low energy states. In MR this is either anti-parallel or parallel to the external magnetic field. The distribution between these two states will be predicted by the Boltzmann equation.

$$N_1/N_2 = \exp(DE/kT)$$

where   N = Number of protons
            DE = Difference in energy levels
            T = Absolute temperature
            k = Boltzmann constant

● **Bandwidth**
The passage of a radiofrequency pulse through tissue will produce signals of varying frequencies. The range of these frequencies is called bandwidth. The image bandwidth must be known before any artifact removal filters are applied to prevent loss or diagnostic signals.

C

● **Carr-Purcell sequence**
T2 characteristics of tissue can be measured by applying a 90 degree RF pulse followed by a train of 180 degree pulses. This results in multiple spin echoes. It is technically difficult to produce perfect 180 degree pulses resulting in "pulse error accumulation". This accumulation can be reduced by altering the 180 degree pulses with reference to one another in 3D space i.e. altering the phase of these pulses in relation to the rotating frame of reference. Such modified sequences are known as Carr-Purcell-Meiboom Gill (CPMG) sequences.

● **Chemical Shift**
This is a misregistration artefact caused by the fact that protons in different parts of a molecule may have slightly different Larmor frequencies due to the "shielding" effect of adjacent bonding electrons. This results in signals from the same voxel being mapped to different pixels causing false signal voids and hyperintensities around the edges of structures or lesions. These effects are exaggerated by higher field strengths and are always seen in the frequency encoded direction. The amount of shift is expressed as parts per million (ppm) of the resonance frequency and is given the greek symbol δ.

Although this is a cause of artefact in imaging it is an important factor in differentiating chemical compounds in spectroscopy (MRS).

Chemical shift selective (CHESS) imaging utilises an RF pulse to saturate only selected compounds before a conventional pulse sequence is used to image the remaining unsaturated compounds. This can be used to differentiate fat from water.

● **CHESS pulses**
A long duration RF pulse has a narrow bandwidth in the frequency domain and can be employed to selectively excite a portion of the spectrum under investigation. These long pulses, typically ~50ms in duration, are called CHESS (Chemical Shift Selective) pulses and are commonly employed in ^1H spectroscopy to suppress the large, unwanted water resonance. CHESS would be used in combination with PRESS or STEAM localisation schemes.

● **Cine-MRI**
Fast image acquisition with sequential looping of the resultant images can be used to display dynamic processes.

Cine-MRI has been particularly useful in cardiology where blood flow can be qualitatively and quantitatively displayed without the need for contrast injection. Joint dynamics such as patellar tracking may also be assessed.

● **Coherence**
Consider the old executive's toy, Newton's Cradle. If all five balls are pulled to one side and then let go, they will all swing together and the motion will continue for some time. This is because they are all swinging in phase and their motion is coherent. But if three balls are pulled to one side and two to the other, the balls will collide and soon cancel their motion out. They have been given opposite phase and their motion lacks coherence. In a similar manner, MR signals from protons in tissue with similar frequency and identical phase are said to be coherent. But proton spin/spin interactions lead to loss of phase coherence and thus the MR signal will decrease with time. This is the basis of T2 relaxation.

● **Coil**
An electric current flowing through a wire will produce a magnetic field around it. Likewise, a changing magnetic field will induce an alternating current in a wire. Specially shaped coils of wire are used in MRI to both produce the RF interrogating pulse and to detect the resultant MR signal from the protons. The voltage strength of these induced currents will be proportional to the MR signal strength.

● **Computer**
The computer is a central component of the MR scanner. It may be used to generate the intrinsic waveforms that must be supplied to each of the gradient amplifiers and to the high power RF amplifier. These waveforms would usually be loaded to some scan controller at the start of an image acquisition thus freeing the computer to allow the display of images and archiving functions to be done in parallel. In-coming signals will have to be digitised prior to manipulation and processing within the computer. Again the scan controller would route these signals to a specialist unit such as an array processor to allow fast processing of images. On completion of the scan and processing the final images would be passed to the more general purpose computer for display.

● **Contrast agents**
The most crucial difference between X-ray and MRI contrast agents is that MRI contrast agents act in an INDIRECT fashion.
X-ray contrast agents work by being directly visible e.g. enhancement is achieved by the increased attenuation of iodine collection in a brain tumour.
In MRI the contrast agents work by altering the relaxation characteristics of the target tissue e.g. enhancement is achieved by gadolinium decreasing the T1 relaxation time of the brain tumour tissue. MR contrast agents may be ferromagnetic, paramagnetic or super paramegnetic.

● **Crosstalk**
Efforts to reduce imaging times in MR resulted in multiple slice acquisition programmes. Unfortunately, unless perfect accuracy is possible, each slice may receive some of the RF pulse intended for adjacent slices which results in degradation of the signal from that slice or spurious echoes. Truly contiguous slices may be obtained by using enhanced spatial encoding incorporated into volume acquisition techniques. Overlapping slices may be acquired by using interleaving sequences which obtain every other slice and then go back to "fill in" the gaps.

● **Cryogen**
Superconducting magnets need to be kept at extremely low temperatures which are maintained by liquified gases or cryogens. The most commonly used are helium (boiling point = $-269\,°C$) and nitrogen (boiling point = $-196\,°C$). These gases tend to boil off over time and can represent a major part of the running costs of a superconducting magnet unless a recycling system is employed. Later magnets use helium-only systems with very low boil-off rates.

D

● **Dead time**
Following an intense RF pulse the delicate receiver electronics are temporarily blinded during the dead time to the true MR signals which are of very low density. The receiver is protected to prevent excessive overload of the system and this may reduce the dead time to be 1 ms (10^{-3}second) or less.

● **Decay time**
After excitation, the protons gradually lose their transverse magnetism (T2) as they precess back to their resting state. The time taken can be referred to as the decay time.

● **DAIR**
The Doubly Attenuated IR sequence combines STIR and FLAIR sequences and can be selected to null signal from fluid and solid structures such as CSF and white matter.

● **Deconvolution**
Deconvolution is the inverse process of convolution. Convolution has a blurring effect upon an image – a single narrow point within an image is transformed to a region of finite width. This occurs for every voxel within the image giving a degraded result. If we know the point spread function, that is exactly how the single narrow point is transformed, then in principle we can invert the process. However, deconvolution is intrinsically unstable in the mathematical sense and is frequently computationally intensive to obtain a satisfactory result.

● **Decoupling**
The term can be employed in two distinct senses, probably of equal importance in NMR.
In the first sense, we are talking about the removal of interaction between the transmitter system and the very sensitive receiver system. This decoupling is required since there is potential for high power transmitter pulses (perhaps peaking at several kilowatts) breaking through into the receiver electronics. The receiver pre-amplifier may be damaged following this overload or the receiver electronics may take some finite time to recover (dead-time). Even when this is not the case there may be a degradation in performance, i.e. a loss of signal-to-noise ratio in resultant images. Decoupling can be achieved by ensuring that the transmitter coil and receiver coil are oriented orthogonally. This is the simplest form of decoupling but is difficult to achieve when coils are of comparable dimensions, complicated design (including the quadrature coil) or is simply anatomically unsuitable. In these cases it is possible to decouple these coils electronically. Decoupling of coils also becomes relevant if there are several receiver coils present simultaneously as in coil array systems.
In the second sense of decoupling we are talking of reducing the inter-nucleur interactions that occur within an assembly of many spins. These interactions can be of magnetic or quadrupolar nature and can be visualised as small perturbations or deviations upon the main static B_0 field. Each nucleus "sees" a slightly different magnetic field dependent upon its environment and a sample responds with a small range of resonant frequencies. The nuclear couplings and their time dependence, caused by random molecular fluctuations, lie at the centre of relaxation phenomena and as a result the subsequent soft tissue contrast observable in MRI. If, for example, proton (^{1}H) signals are broadened by ^{1}H neighbours then we have homonuclear coupling. When broadened by other magnetic nuclei such as carbon (^{13}C) it is known as heternuclear coupling. Decoupling techniques developed on classical NMR spectroscopy have been applied to *in vivo* MRS phosphorus (^{31}P) and ^{13}C studies in recent years where ^{1}H is the offending, coupled nucleus. Decoupling techniques involve the systematic and repeated inversion of the nuclei causing the broadening while receiving the signal from the spins under investigation. As such decoupling requires additional radio-frequency pulses, with a commensurate increase in potential absorption by the patient.

● **DRESS**
This is an early spectroscopic localisation technique that uses a surface coil and a slice selective pulse to define a planar region from which signal can be derived. Depth Resolved Surface Spectroscopy or DRESS has been used extensively in the past to acquire ^{31}P spectra. A slice interleaved version, known as SLIT-DRESS and using the same logic as multi-slice imaging, allows more efficient use of scan time to acquire more spectroscopic data.

● **Detector**
In MR the detector is a small coil or loop of copper wire. Additional capacitors make the detector a resonant circuit which is tuned to the Larmor frequency for the nuclei under investigation. The signal is predominantly this single frequency (in whole body systems 1-100MHz) but there are small variations due to unintentional magnetic field imperfections (in range 10-100s Hz), the deliberate applications of imaging gradient fields (range ±10s kHz) and inter-nuclear coupling (10s Hz). The demodulator strips out the main Larmor frequency (MHz), known as the carrier, leaving the small variations at low or audio frequencies (kHz). This remnant lower frequency signal is the free induction decay that is usually drawn in the textbooks.

● **Dewar**
This is the name given to an insulted container for the storage of cryogens. These are bulky and consideration must be given to their access to the magnet room when designing an MR facility.

● **Diamagnetic**
If a substance placed in a magnetic field becomes magnetised in the opposite direction to that field, it will cause a localised decrease in the field and is said to have diamagnetic properties or negative susceptibility.

● **Diffusion**
Random thermal motion of molecules results in their intermingling over time. MR can provide a sensitive technique for measuring the diffusion of some substances which can be utilised to provide tissue characterisation.

● **Dipole**
When two small electric charges of opposite sign are physically displaced with respect to one another then an electric dipole is created. On the other hand a magnetic dipole is created by a simple current carrying loop. A spinning, singly charged atomic nucleus is viewed in classical physics as a current loop and as such has an associated magnetic moment or nuclear bar magnet with a north and south pole. This classical picture fails since the neutron (electrically uncharged) has a magnetic moment and not all charged nuclei have nuclear dipoles e.g. ^{12}C is NMR-invisible while ^{13}C (1.1% abundant) can be detected. The difference is due to the arrangement of nucleons (protons and neutrons) within the nucleus.

Small bar magnets have dipolar fields which extend into the surrounding region – remember those iron filings of years ago! These cause nuclei to interact or couple together and it is possible to talk of a local field at a particular nucleus due to its neighbours. The static or time independent part to this local field broadens MR resonances i.e. is related to the T_2 of a spin system. The time dependent portion of the local field effects **both** T_1 and T_2 processes.

● **Dispersion**
The rate of relaxation of tissue will alter at different strengths of the external magnetic field (B_0). This variation is known as dispersion and it is an important quantity in the study of relaxation mechanics. Knowledge of dispersion profiles is important in the development of MR contrast agents.

- **Display Matrix**
This refers to the number of picture elements (pixels) which form each line of the image. A typical high quality image will have 512 pixels per line and 512 pixels per column – a "512 × 512" image. However, in order to see a high quality image, the acquisition matrix must equal or succeed that of the display matrix. If the display matrix is greater than the acquisition matrix then data are repeated in adjacent pixels by a process known as interpolation. The final image would therefore lack detail.

- **Dixon Technique**
Water and fat signals are separated by a small amount in frequency terms due to chemical shift, a coupling that is proportional to the strength of the applied static field B_0. This results, particularly at higher field strengths, to the chemical shift artefact – a black voxel where the water and fat content are very nearly equal and are in anti-phase (and cancel). These black voxels give a delineated appearance, a contour of voxels where water and fat equate. Dixon's method, acquiring two images with differing echo times, allows the separation of water and fat as two distinct images. Neither image will have the chemical shift artefact thus exposing anything of underlying interest.

- **Duty cycle**
A MRI scanner has pulsed RF and pulsed gradient systems. The duty cycle is the fraction of time "on" to the fraction "off"; 100% represents continuous usage. Multi-slice capability has a requirement for a higher duty cycle. This in turn requires systems such as amplifiers to be capable of delivering power for greater fractions of time and coils to be able to dissipate this power as heat.

E

- **Echo**
The echo phenomenon in MR takes two distinct forms – the field or gradient reversal echo and the spin echo. The field echo is more sensitive to magnetic field inhomogeneities than the spin echo and as such is less flattering in terms of good looking images. On the other hand its susceptibility to field imperfections can be exploited clinically e.g. investigations of haemorrhage.

Field echoes are formed by the reversal of the imaging gradient during which magnetisation, which can be viewed as precessing in a clockwise direction (say) initially, is simply unwound in the anti-clockwise direction following the gradient reversal. Inhomogeneities are **not** reversed since they are attached, or due to magnet, or the patient and the precession will be in only one direction. If the field is very bad then signal losses occur within a single vortex of an image due to the phase cancellation of spins.

Spin echoes involve two RF pulses; a 90° pulse followed a few tens of milliseconds later by a 180° pulse. Precessional direction is not reversed by the second pulse but rather it is advanced; slower spins initially lagging are put closer to the "finish", the echo time TE, than the faster spins. They all rephase at twice the pulse separation (TE) to give a spin echo which is reduced in amplitude because of non-reversible relaxation processes and diffusive phenomena.

- **Echo planar imaging**
EPI is a fast imaging technique requiring high gradient usage and fast signal sampling rates. There is a strain on the gradient amplifier system and eddy currents for faster imaging techniques including multi-slice methods.

The EPI technique involves rapidly switching the frequency encode gradient (a series of field echoes) and incrementing the phase encoding during a single free induction decay. Since the rate of data acquisition is high the bandwidth of the system must be broader and this introduces more noise. To date the loss in signal-to-noise has been compensated for by the increase in voxel size i.e. a loss in spatial resolution. The process is virtually real-time and offers the prospect of interactive MR at the cost of increased RF energy deposition in the patient. The rapid rate of change of the magnetic gradients can also cause peripheral nerve stimulation, although the switching rates now used in image formation do not cause observable effects.

● **Eddy currents**
Any conductor in a changing magnetic field will develop eddy currents; these currents develop their own magnetic fields which are in opposition to the original change. Eddy currents prevent rapid rates of changes in the gradient system and therefore are the bane of the fast imagers' life. Without compensation of some sort they cause image degradation even with more conventional multi-slice 2DFT MRI. In recent years self-shielding gradient coils have been developed in order to reduce the coupling (again) between the coils and the magnet bore.

● **Electromagnetic Radiation**
This is the transmission of energy by variations in electric and magnetic fields in the form of waves. The frequency of the waveform gives the radiation its physical properties. Radio, visible light and X-rays are merely electromagnetic radiation at different frequencies.

● **Electron**
These negatively charged particles have a mass of only 1/1850th of a proton. However, they have an important contribution to the magnetic resonance frequency of the nucleus as their orbital path around the nucleus is associated with a small magnetic field which "shields" the nucleus from external magnetic fields. This "shielding" effect is the phenomenon of chemical shift.

● **Enhancement**
MRI contrast media enhance in an indirect fashion by altering the relaxation rate of the target tissue. Intravascular contrast agents such as Gadolinium have the same pharmacological distribution as conventional IV contrast media but the change in image contrast is due to alteration of the physical properties of the target tissue and not the presence of the contrast agent itself.

● **Ernst Angle**
Fast scanning techniques utilising low flip angles (i.e. less than 90 degrees) can suffer from reduced signal from the sample volume. In an effort to maximise the signal the optimum flip angle for the tissue under study can be used. This is known as the Ernst Angle.

● **Even Echo Rephasing**
In multi-echo imaging sequences, rephasing gradients are selected to give optimal rephasing of spins (and therefore the best signal) on even multiples of the original Time to Echo (TE), e.g. 2TE, 4TE and so on. It can be shown that nuclei changing position linearly in the time are refocussed exactly at the even echo it regardless of their exact velocity.

● **Excitation**
In order to generate an MR signal from tissue, its component spins must have energy put into them. This is done by the interrogating or exciting radiofrequency pulse.

F

● Faraday Cage
To prevent the effects of stray or unwanted radio frequencies from outside affecting the transmit/receive coils a cage of conducting material (usually copper) must be placed around the machine.

● Fast Imaging
Various techniques such as reducing the flip angle and using gradient echoes have been developed to try and overcome the inherently slow image formation time in MRI. A large number of acronyms have sprung up, many the result of different companies giving the same technique a different name. FLASH, FISP, GRASS and RARE are some of the more familiar acronyms.

● Fat Suppression
Signal from tissue protons consists of water and fat components. Various imaging sequences have been devised to null that part of the signal arising from fat (such as Short Tau Inversion Recovery or STIR), leaving an image showing the distribution of water. This is useful for delineating tissue that is oedematous as a result of inflammation, infection or tumour involvement.

● Ferromagnetic
Any substance which has a large positive magnetic susceptibility and an ability to retain residual magnetisation is termed a ferromagnetic substance. An essential physical property of such substances is that they contain microscopic volumes or "domains" in which there are unpaired electron spins. In a non-magnetised state these domains are randomly orientated, but after exposure to an external magnetic field the domains align with one another, and remain aligned after removal of the external field. This alignment will result in the substance demonstrating its own intrinsic magnetism.

● Field Strength
Referred to equations as B_0, the field strength is a measure of the magnitude of the external magnetic field provided by the imaging system and is given in Teslas (T). In clinical imaging the field strength is often referred to as low, medium or high. Low field strengths range from 0.02 to 0.3T, medium field strengths from 0.3 to 1.0T and any systems operating above 1.0T are referred to as high field. Imaging nuclei other than hydrogen requires field strengths of 1.5T or greater owing to their inferior sensitivity. High field is also required to increase the chemical shift dispersion such that individual resonances of an MR spectrum can be resolved.

● Field of View (FOV)
This is the product of the acquisition matrix used and the pixel dimensions or resolution in the final image. Adapting the field of view to the size of the part under study is an important method in reducing aliasing (wraparound). Decreasing the FOV improves spectral resolution at the expense of reducing the signal to noise ratio.

● Filling Factor
The achievement of optimal signal-to-noise ratios in MR images depends in part on efficient RF irradiation and signal detection which requires a close fit between the transmit/receive coils and the part under study. The efficiency of this fit can be expressed as the geometrical relationship between the coil and the part (volume of part/volume of coil) and is termed the filling factor.

● Filtering
Signal processing to remove noise or aliasing artifacts can be achieved by altering the frequency content by a process known as filtering. The signal in its electrical form can be filtered by standard analogue devices or numerical algorithms can be applied to digitised data.

● **FISP**
A fast imaging acronym that stands for Fast Imaging with Steady State Free Precession. The steady state free precession of spins is achieved by applying a train of RF pulses with interpulse intervals much shorter than T2. The signals from 2 consecutive pulses are then observed together to provide image information. Main field inhomogeneities and imperfect gradients are significant detractors from image quality with this technique.

● **FLAIR**
The Fluid Attenuated Inversion Recovery or FLAIR sequence has an Inversion Time (TI) selected to allow the nulling of the signals from image components having a long T_1 such as CSF and other fluids.

● **FLASH**
A commonly used acronym standing for Fast Low Angle Shot. This is a fast imaging technique that employs a reduced flip angle to maintain signal-to-noise ratio and manipulate image contrast. The sequence will run at TR of below 100ms and data acquisition periods are very short.

● **Flip Angle**
This is a measure of the amount of rotation of the bulk magnetic vector of the tissue under study away from the axis of the main magnetic field (B_0) produced by the interrogating RF pulse. The amount of flip is proportional to the amplitude and duration of the RF pulse, this product is proportional to the energy in the pulse.

● **Flow Artifacts**
Both artifactual signal voids (time of flight signal loss) and hyperintense areas (flow related enhancement) can be caused by flow phenomena in body fluids. Flowing matter can take signal away from an area of data acquisition to cause a void and it can equally bring signal into an area from adjacent excitations in multi-slice acquisitions. Such flow-related enhancements occur more readily with rapid sequences and on multi-slice MRI. Flow artifacts can be reduced by using pre-saturation pulses which "de-magnetise" the protons which are about to flow into the image volume.

● **FOLD**
A functional MRI mechanism that is FlOw Level Dependent. This theorises that the increase in regional blood flow causes the observable signal change in activated neural tissue.

● **Fourier Transform**
This is a mathematical tool which is used to convert the raw MR signal into its frequency and phase components. In multiple-slice imaging, frequency and phase define the x and y co-ordinate system for the final image. Hence a 2 dimensional Fourier transformation will be sufficient (2-DFT). However, if data have been acquired from a volume rather than a slice then a third co-ordinate will be needed which requires a third Fourier transformation (3-DFT). Further if spectroscopic data is acquired a fourth dimension is added (4-DFT or 4D-CSI).

● **Free Induction Decay (FID)**
When a gyroscope is tipped away from its vertical spinning axis it will return to its upright position in a spiralling motion and the amount of this precession around its axis will decay with a characteristic time constant. In the same way a spinning proton tipped from the main magnetic field of an MR magnet by the interrogating RF pulse will return to alignment with the main magnetic field (in time constant T2★). During this time the MRI signal from this proton will decay from the maximum at 90 degrees to the main field to zero when parallel to the field. This decaying signal is called the Free Induction Decay.

● **Frequency and Encoding**
In a flat plane any point on that plane can be described by its x and y co-ordinates. In a 2-D MRI image slice the equivalent of the x and y co-ordinates are the frequency and phase characteristics of each point. If the x scale is to be the "frequency" characteristics then a range of frequency values across the slice must be provided by "encoding" the MR signals from protons along that slice. This is done by applying a magnetic gradient along the slice so that each point experiences a unique additional magnetic field. Since the frequency of precession of the spins is proportional to the magnetic field at each point, a frequency range will exist along the slice allowing the "x" co-ordinate for each point to be determined.

● **Functional Imaging (fMRI)**
Functional Imaging refers to a collection of methods that have been developed to study regional brain activity. They all make use of a common principle: the utilisation of oxygen by activated neural tissue. This utilization will affect the proportion of oxy- and deoxyhaemaglobin and also alter the regional blood flow. These changes will affect the homogeneity of the local magnetic field in the area of activation. T2★ weighted sequences (such as gradient echo and echo planar) will be sensitive to the homogeneity changes and can thus image the activation zone. As usual, the mechanisms thought to be involved have been given catchy acronyms, such as BOLD and FOLD.

G

● **Gadolinium**
The first clinically available contrast medium for MRI was the chelate of this metal from the Lanthanide series with diethylenetriamine penta-acetic acid (DTPA). The ion of gadolinium has the greatest paramagnetic effect due to the number of unpaired electrons but is highly toxic in the unbound state. Its chelation provides safe bio-availability without removing its paramagnetic properties.

● **Gating**
In order to remove the effects of physiologic motion from tissues or fluids MR data can be acquired at the same point in each motion cycle. Successful gating requires regular or cyclical motion. Thus gating cannot overcome artifact due to bowel movement. Another problem is that gating techniques can often add significantly to imaging time. This has been a particular problem in the upper abdomen where the effects of both cardiac and respiratory motion have to be overcome.

● **Gauss**
A Gauss (G) is a unit of magnetic flux density. This has been replaced in the SI system by the Tesla (T), where 1T = 10,000G. The Gauss is still used as a convenient method of annotating very small fields such as the stray field around an MR system.

● **Ghost Artifact**
Pulsatile flow produces complex multi-layered bands of high signal propagated in the phase encoded direction. Although usually the result of vascular pulsation, CSF flow, cardiac motion and body wall motion will also cause ghosting. The effects of this artifact are more prominent in longer imaging sequences. If the artifact interferes with diagnosis the phase encoding direction can be altered or gating techniques can be employed. Sometimes the artifact can be useful, for example as in identifying vessels in complex regions such as the thoracic inlet.

● **Gradients**
In order to localise MR signals emanating from protons in 3 dimensions a series of 3 magnetic field gradients are superimposed on the external magnetic field (Bo). This results in each point in a volume of tissue experiencing a unique magnetic field strength. Thus the Larmour frequency of precession will be unique for each point which allows for selective excitation or detection. The 3 gradients are:

Slice selection gradient
Phase encoding gradient
Frequency gradient.

● **Gradient Echo Imaging**
Spin-Echo imaging achieves T2-weighting by nullifying the effects of the magnetic field inhomogeneities with a 180 degree "rephasing" pulse. Unfortunately this tactic increases TE and increases the amount of RF power deposited in tissues. However, T2-weighting can also be achieved by rapid reversals of the read-out gradients and acquiring the resultant echoes. The contrast in these images are dependent on the T2★ signal (the sum of T2 and the effects of magnetic field inhomogeneities) and so they are sensitive to unstable or impure static fields. Image acquisition time is reduced both by the deletion of the 180 degree rephasing pulse and by the ability to reduce flip angles owing to the rapidity with which gradient reversals can be applied.

H

● **h**
In quantum mechanics electromagnetic radiation is composed of small packets or quanta. The energy E of each quantum is related to its frequency ν by the equation

$$E = h\nu$$

where h is Planck's constant. h has the value of 6.626×10^{-34} Js (Joule second). The energy of quanta of rf radiation is extremely small when compared to molecular bonding which underpins the belief in the intrinsic safety of magnetic resonance.

● **H**
H is the symbol for magnetic field intensity. It has the units of Amperes/metre in the SI system. The magnetic induction B within a material, which would determine the exact Larmor frequency, is dependent upon its magnetic properties, encapsulated by the relative permeability μ_r, is related to H by the equation

$$B = \mu_r \mu_0 H$$

where μ_0 is the permeability of a vacuum, which has a value of $4\pi \times 10^{-7}$ Henry/metre. μ_r is less than 1 for a diamagnetic material and greater than 1 for a paramagnetic substance. Materials which are ferromagnetic such as iron have very large values of μ_r.

● **Homogeneity**
The Larmor equation, relating the frequency ν to the magnetic induction B within a sample,

$$\nu = \gamma B$$

emphasises that there is a great premium to be had by having a very good quality or homogeneous magnetic field. Highly homogeneous fields will ensure that the resonance is achieved over very narrow band of frequencies. The basic magnet quality is improved by the process of shimming. The final quality is expressed in parts per million (ppm). It is important to note the volume from which the homogeneity figure is derived, typically a 30-40 cm sphere, when comparisons are being made. Local deviations in field homogeneity can result from metallic implants, shunts and the like. They may also occur at tissue interfaces and in haemorrhagic regions. The effect of these local field deviations in the first instance is to dephase the MR signal and cause signal reductions. In severe examples the image can be distorted in appearance.

The homogeneity of the B_1 field is also important since it is required that all the specified pulses are applied to the whole volume of interest. If this is not the case then there are spatial variations in contrast.

I

● **I**

The spin angular momentum of an atomic nucleus is denoted by the symbol I. I is measured in units of ℏ (which represents the value of Planck's constant (h) divided by 2π) and can take any multiple of 1/2. A nucleus that is spinning also has as a magnetic moment whose size is dependent upon the magnetogyric ratio (γ) which is constant for a given isotope.

Spin angular momentum is a vector quantity, that has x, y and z-components and therefore has a magnitude and direction. The magnitude is given by $\sqrt{I(I+1)}$. Quantum mechanics demand that nuclear spins can only assume certain orientations when placed in a magnetic field B_0. There are 2I+1 quantised states each labelled by the symbol m_I, the nuclear spin quantum number. Each of these orientations has a different energy in B_0. The m_I can take the values +I, I-1, . . . -I which equate to an allowed component of the nuclear magnetic moment along the direction of B_0. By convention this quantised direction is labelled the z-axis. The other two components (in this case x and y) are not constrained in any way by quantum mechanics. Classically each nuclear magnet can be envisaged as precessing at an angle to the main static field B_0. Since m_I can never equate to the magnitude of the angular momentum a nuclear spin can never align perfectly along the applied field.

The nucleus of principal interest in MRI, the proton or ^1H, has the spin value of 1/2. In this case the magnitude of the angular momentum is $\sqrt{3}/2$ and there are two m_I states with the values -1/2 and +1/2.

Phosphorus (^{31}P) carbon (^{13}C) and fluorine (^{19}F) also have a spin angular momentum of 1/2. On the other hand deuterium (^2H) has a spin of 1 while sodium (^{23}Na) takes the value of 5/2. Nuclei with zero spin are invisible from the MR point of view; the abundant isotope of carbon (^{12}C) falls into this category, as does ^{16}O.

● **Induction**

The term induction is used in two senses in MR, not entirely unrelated, but worthy of distinct explanation.

a) Magnetic field strength is denoted by the symbol H and has the units of amperes/metre. Any object inserted into this field will have a magnetic flux induced within it. Magnetic induction, denoted by the symbol B, has the units of Tesla. The extent of the magnetic induction is dependent upon the magnetic permeability (μ) of the material which is usually compared to the value for free space (μ_0). NMR texts are phenomenally bad in switching between H and B and interchanging the units of B and H. Strictly we should be concerned with the magnetic induction B since this will depend upon the nature of the material or body within the field H.

b) A constant current passed through a wire loop generates a magnetic field along the axis of that loop. This is the basis upon which the static field B_0 is generated. The converse, that a magnetic field applied to a coil generates a current, is **not** true. In order to generate any current in the coil the magnetic field must be varying in time and this is an expression of Faraday's law of magnetic induction. Strictly it is required that the magnetic flux cutting through the conducting loop vary in time in order to generate a time varying current. Transverse magnetisation and its associated magnetic flux lines precess at the Larmor frequency with respect to the magnet and receive coil. A time dependent current is induced, with the small variations in precessional frequency being reflected by commensurate changes in current in the receiver coil. This signal is subsequently amplified prior to digitisation and further processing within a computer.

● **Inhomogeneity**

The term inhomogeneity can be applied to the applied static field B_0 and the radio frequency (rf) or B_1 fields employed in MR. In each case the quality of the respective magnetic field over the extent of the imaged region is of relevance.

The local magnetic field can be varying due to spatial variations caused by imperfections or inhomogeneities in B_0. A magnet system system would usually have some corrective mechanism, called shimming, that allows field imperfections to be reduced. This procedure would be done at the time of installation of the magnet and would not require further attention as long as the environment of the magnet was not changed significantly.

Magnetic fields also vary due to inter-nuclear interactions that are intrinsic to the materials and tissues that are being observed. In a perfect world one would like the inhomogeneity of B_0 to be less than these intrinsic line broadening mechanisms within the sample being studied with MR.

MR images require that the sample or body be irradiated with rf fields in order to generate the signal. Rf pulse sequences are employed in order to manipulate image contrast. We can see that it is required that the rf pulses are constant across the whole imaging plane. If this is not the case then there will be spatial variations in image contrast due to inhomogeneities in the radio frequency or B_1 field.

The attributes or receiver coil inhomogeneity are usually less subtle than those of the transmitter coil and are identified by fall-off in image intensity.

● Interleaving

This is a method of reducing scanning times by acquiring more than one slice at a time. Selecting and encoding a slice may only take 50msec, but the TR may be much longer to allow image contrast to develop. However, it is possible to utilise this "wait time" to obtain data from other slice locations in an interleaved fashion.

● Inversion time (TI)

The interval TI denotes the interval between 180° inversion pulse and subsequent 90° observation pulse in an inversion-recovery pulse sequence. TI may be manipulated to wall signals with specific T_1; STIR is employed to suppress fat, FLAIR to reduce signal from CSF.

● Inversion-recovery sequence (IR)

The IR sequence is specifically employed to measure the longitudinal magnetisation following an initial 180° pulse. If a series of inversion recovery sequences are employed this can allow the relaxation behaviour of the longitudinal magnetisation to be measured and its associated time constant T_1 calculated. In MRI it is simply employed as a means of emphasising T_1 by selecting a single TI.

As its name implies the sequence commences with a 180° or inversion rf pulse. It is usually assumed that the nuclear spins are all aligned along B_0 prior to this pulse. As a result there is no signal directly after the perfect inversion pulse since no transverse components of magnetisation are generated. The magnetisation is rotated from +z to -z. Following the inversion the nuclei are free to re-establish themselves as they please which will be to restore their orientations with respect to the magnet. The longitudinal component of magnetisation becomes less negative, passes through zero and heads towards +z. Since longitudinal magnetisation can not be seen directly we must apply an observing 90° pulse to take a look at the extent of the relaxation along B_0. The 90° pulse occurs a time TI after the 180° or inversion pulse. This "look" can involve the imaging gradients to allow the construction of an image if required. The resultant image will contain a heavy weighting toward the T_1 process.

Since the magnetisation along the field can lie in the range -z to +z there is potentially double the range of magnetisation to manipulate and there is scope to generate images with greater contrast. Best contrast occurs in the region when longitudinal magnetisation is close to zero as it passes from -z to +z. This is because at this point in the relaxation recovery the change of longitudinal magnetisation is at its greatest. Inversion-recovery scans are apt to look noisy although contrast is good. IR imaging sequences are usually amongst the slower scans since TR is usually 1.5 seconds or longer. However the scope to manipulate contrast to a greater extent and to allow the nulling of troublesome hyper-intense signals as in the Short TI Inversion Recovery (STIR) sequence gives these sequences considerable usage.

● **ISIS – Image Selected *In-vivo* Spectroscopy**
ISIS consists of three orthogonal slice selective 180° pulses in combination with a phase cycling scheme. The phase cycling and data accumulation required introduces a minimum of eight transients before the volume localised spectrum can be observed. The technique has been extended to include the multiple acquisition of several voxels simultaneously, and conformation of the voxel shape to match required pathological regions, ISIS and its developments have been applied extensively to ^{31}P MRS. It is less useful in ^{1}H spectroscopy since the eight required transients cover a large dynamic range of signal strengths.

● **Isotope**
Atoms of the same element but having different masses. This means they have the same number of protons, i.e. atomic number but differing numbers of neutrons within the nucleus of the atom. From a MR point of view a number of rules apply:

(a) Isotopes of even mass number and even charge have zero spin – as examples, ^{12}C, ^{16}O, ^{32}S.

(b) Isotopes of even mass number and odd charge have integral spin $-^2$H, ^{14}N.

(c) Isotopes of odd mass number have half-integral spin $-^1$H, ^{3}H, ^{19}F, ^{13}C, ^{23}Na.

J

● **J**
The symbol J is employed to denote the strength of the J or scalar coupling interaction between nuclei. It has the units of frequency (Hertz).

● **J-coupling**
Also known as scalar coupling is a basic interaction between two magnetic spins. From an NMR point of view both spins may be of a nuclear origin or alternatively one may be of an electronic nature. The latter of these, the nuclear-electron interaction, can be a potent source of relaxation nuclear spins when the electron is periodically re-orienting as a result of its own relaxation or due to the mobility of the molecule to which it is attached.

Scalar coupling, like the dipolar interaction between nuclei, is independent of the field strength B_0 which contrast with the chemical shift effect which varies linearly with B_0. However, unlike the dipolar interaction, the J-coupling between nuclei does not average to zero as the nuclei tumble around in the liquid state. Scalar couplings are observed in spectroscopy when resonances are split into multiplet patterns. The observed splittings are usually small, say 1-10 Hertz, and are usually observed as small deviations upon the chemical shift interaction. To date there has been little impact or usage of the J-coupling of spins in MRI.

K

● **k**
The symbol for the fundamental constant known as Boltzmann's constant. The constant arises in statistical mechanics which draws together the quantum mechanical behaviour of small particles such as molecules and atoms into large scale macroscopically measurable properties.

● **Kilo**
Prefix denoting 1000, as in kHz meaning 1000Hz.

● **K-Space**
K-Space is an imaginary mathematical space into which the raw data from phase and frequency encoding is built up to form a raw data matrix. The points at the centre of this space contribute to image contrast whereas the points nearer the edges give spatial resolution.
In conventional spin echo imaging one line of K-space is filled per pulse repetition cycle. Fast spin echo techniques can be achieved by using echo trains to fill more than one line of K-space per repetition cycle.

L

● **Larmor frequency**
A nuclear magnet, when placed in a magnetic field, can be visualised as precessing in the manner of a spinning top. The rate at which this precession occurs is known as the Larmor frequency. From a quantum mechanical viewpoint the nuclear magnetic moment is contrained to have only a discrete set of energies when in the magnetic field. The energy difference between these quantized levels matches the classical Larmor frequency. (See also Homogeneity).

● **Lineshape**
An isolated nuclear spin in a perfect magnetic field would resonate at a single frequency and this would be represented as an infinitely narrow spike in the frequency spectrum. This simplistic picture is disturbed by inter-nuclear interactions and by inhomogeneities in the applied field. In both cases the frequency spectrum has a finite width and the infinitely narrow spike in reality has some lineshape. The NMR lineshape is often fitted to bell-shaped mathematical forms such as the Lorentzian or Gaussian functions. Analysis of lineshapes can give structural information but the principal is hampered by the realities of imperfect magnetic fields and susceptibility effects caused by the sample itself. A variety of techniques are available to reduce these latter effects not least of all the spin echo which has received widespread usage in MRI.

● **Localisation**
In order to generate a useful image spatial localisation is required to limit the regions from which MR signals are received. In mainstream MRI, by which we mean multi-slice planar imaging, the principle components of signal localisation are the slice selection process followed by the subsequent frequency and phase encoding on the resultant excited signal.

● **Longitudinal magnetisation (M_0, M_z)**
Individual nuclear magnets precess freely when placed in a magnetic field B_0. In a classical description these magnetic moments have components that are longitudinal to the B_0 field (by convention taken to be the z-axis) but also have transverse (x and y components). However quantum mechanics demands that the z-component is limited to a small number of values. Each orientation has a different energy and lower energies are very marginally preferred. According to statistical mechanics this orientational preference represents only 1 spin in 100000. There is a net component oriented along the field B_0 as a result of all these unbalanced spins and this constitutes the longitudinal magnetisation. We should note that the large numbers of nuclei involved ensure that the transverse components of individual precessing nuclei cancel out.
At thermal equilibrium, by which we mean a long time after putting the subject in the field or after any rf pulses, there is only the longitudinal component of nuclear magnetisation and this is given the symbol M_0. M_z is a more generalised symbol for the longitudinal magnetisation that reflects the fact that it may not be at equilibrium. In the long run M_z will fully relax to the value of M_0.

Longitudinal magnetisation can not be observed directly by MR. The conventional receiver coil will pick-up transverse magnetisation only since they are precessing and will induce measurable currents. The state of the magnetisation along the B_0 field is monitored with a 90° rf pulse whose effect is simply to rotate the z-component into transverse plane (xy) where it can be observed.

● **Longitudinal relaxation**
Relaxation of magnetisation along the direction of the static applied field B_0. Following an excitatory rf pulse, during which energy is put into the spin system and the imbalance of populations between the allowed energy states is disturbed, individual nuclei re-orient themselves with respect to the B_0 field. The longitudinal magnetisation changes in time as relaxation processes restore the system to its equilibrium state. As this relaxation or reorientation takes place there is a loss in spin-energy and this is conceptually given up to a lattice, other degrees of freedom within the sample that can dissipate the energy, hence its other name of spin-lattice relaxation. The process of longitudinal relaxation is given the time-constant of T_1. Over any period of T_1, during which there is no interference upon the nuclear spin system, a 63% recovery of the longitudinal magnetisation will take place. In the first T_1 63% recovery occurs, in the next T_1 63% of the remaining 37% recovers and so on. It is usually assumed that after five repetitions ($5 \times T_1$) complete relaxation has taken place.
Longitudinal relaxation can be measured with the use of the inversion-recovery sequence.

M

● **Magic Angle**
Body structures composed of a linear sub-structure, such as the collagen fibrils in ligaments, tendons and cartilege, may undergo paradoxical signal increase when the linear axis subtends an angle of 55° to the main magnet field, B_0. The appearances are most noticeable on T_1 weighted images and where tendons and cartilege have a curved path such as in the shoulder and ankle.

● **Magnet**
The magnet is the central piece of equipment of the MR scanner. It should provide a field (B_0) whose strength is stable over a period of time and spatially homogeneous over a region that must compare in size with the object to be imaged. The homogeneity is expressed as a parts per million (ppm) figure for a defined volume of space, say a 30 or 50 cm diameter sphere.
Magnets may be permanent, resistive or superconducting in construction. For higher fields, above 2.0T, the superconducting magnets present the only choice. Permanent magnets are built from blocks of ferromagnetic alloys of metals such as nickel, iron and cobalt. The source of ferromagnetism is the unpaired electrons within the component elements of these alloys. Resistive magnets consist of many windings of copper wire and the field is maintained by the permanent supply of electrical current from a suitably stabilised power supply. Superconducting magnets are similar in the respect of having many windings. However, rather than copper, alloys of metals such as niobium and tin are employed whose characteristic is that they lose all electrical resistance when reduced in temperature. Once energised a superconducting magnet will maintain a field without additional power consumption. The catch is that incredibly low temperatures have to be maintained usually in the region of 20K (20° above absolute zero [approximately -273°C]). The electricity bill is replaced by the expense of the cryogenic (cooling) gases nitrogen and helium, although many magnets now require helium only.
MRI is carried out in fields ranging from 0.1T to 1.5T with a preponderance at 0.5T and above. Magnetic resonance spectroscopy (MRS) requires high field strength and for whole body *in vivo* work this usually equates to 1.5T although proton (^1H) MRS has been demonstrated at 1.0T.

● **Magnetic moment**
Magnetic moment is a descriptive term employed interchangeably with, for example, nuclear spin, nuclear magnet or nucleus.

A conventional bar magnet will align itself with a magnetic field, a concept we are familiar with in the compass. The magnetic moment is strictly defined as the force required to keep the bar magnet or compass needle at right angles to this preferred alignment along the field. The greater the strength of the bar magnet or field, the greater the magnetic moment.

The *nuclear* magnetic moment when placed in a magnetic field can take only a small number of orientations and can never perfectly align itself along this field. The energy differences between these orientations are the basis of the magnetic resonance phenomenon. The size of the nuclear magnetic moment is directly proportional to the magnetogyric ratio of the element (or more specifically isotope) under investigation.

● **Magnetic interactions**
These interactions or couplings are the basis for the MR phenomenon. Time independent or motionally averaged interactions determine the positions of nuclear resonances in the frequency spectrum. Fluctuating or time dependent magnetic couplings, particularly when they are varying at a rate close to the Larmor frequency, have a significant role in the relaxation of the nuclei under investigation.

The primary magnetic interaction is between the applied magnetic field (B_0) and the nuclear magnetic moment, the nuclear Zeeman effect. The size of this interaction is dependent upon the B_0 field strength and would be most commonly expressed as the Larmor frequency that lies in the range 5-64 MHz for the whole body MRI systems. Superimposed upon this Zeeman interaction are much smaller interactions between nuclei and the electrons within their immediate environment and between the magnetic nuclei themselves. All of these interactions are of the order of a million times smaller than the Zeeman coupling. In order to see them it is perhaps not unreasonable to seek magnets that are accurate or homogeneous to this one-millionth degree, that is a part per million (ppm). This is not always possible but there are MR techniques, such as the spin echo, that compensate for the lack of homogeneity to the required level.

● **Magnetogyric ratio, γ**
The magnetogyric ratio (γ) relates the magnetic field strength (B) to the nuclear precessional or Larmor frequency (ω). This is summarised by the Larmor equation.

$$\omega = \gamma B$$

Note that ω is the angular frequency which is simply the usual Larmor frequency expressed in Hertz multiplied by 2π.

● **Magnetisation**
Magnetisation is the bulk equivalent of magnetic moment and is defined as the density of magnetic moment per unit volume (of tissue in clinical MR). There are various contributions to the overall magnetisation induced when a body is placed in a magnetic field. These include the diamagnetism of the electrons and the paramagnetism of the nuclei.

Nuclear magnetisation is generated by the alignment of atomic nuclei within the applied field. It represents one of the smaller components of the total magnetisation.

The induced magnetisation (M) generated is proportional to field (B) and this is expressed by the equation.

$$M = \chi B$$

where χ is the (nuclear) susceptibility and will vary between tissues. Unlike individual nuclear magnetic moments the magnetisation can align perfectly along the applied magnetic. Intuitively it can be imagined that the individual spins contributing to the magnetisation are all precessing at essentially the same frequency but at random phases with respect to one another.

Without being too strict the basic magnetisation of a tissue can be equated to the proton density, it defines the amount of signal that can be generated. This is not really true since MRI observable nuclei are only those more mobile protons within a tissue whose longitudinal relaxation time T_1 are not too long and transverse times T_2 not too short. Amongst soft tissues the variation in intrinsic magnetisation is not so great. Contrast is greatly improved by exploiting variations in relaxation times between tissues.

● **Magnetisation Transfer Contrast (MTC)**
Contrast between soft tissues can be increased by exploring the fact that there is an interaction between mobile hydrogen protons in water and restricted protons in macromolecules or immobile water.
The T_2 of bound protons is so far short that they are not usually seen in MR images. However, the interaction between bound and mobile protons still exists and it will be influenced if one or other type is saturated by an on-off resonance pulse.
Thus, by saturating the bound proton pool, the contrast of the mobile proton pool can be manipulated. This can be exploited to improve contrast between normal and diseased tissue or to amplify the effect of a contrast agent.

● **Maximum Intensity Projection**
A computer generated reformatting technique that displays only the highest signals along lines drawn through an imaging plane. When all the imaging planes are summated a 3D representation of the highest signal structures can be generated. The commonest application is in MR Angiography where pulse sequences are used which produce the highest signal in thin blood vessels. The final "MIPPED" images will then give a 3D representation of the signal from flowing blood free of background tissue.

● **Mega-**
In metric units the prefix mega- is employed to denote one million times and is usually abbreviated to M. Hence 1MHz becomes one million Hertz.

● **MESA – Multiple Echo Spectroscopic Acquisition**
MESA is a spin echo based spectroscopic localisation technique that employs three mutually orthogonal slice selective 180° pulses to define to a given region of interest. Initial transverse magnetisation is generated by a binomial excitation where the large water resonance remains along the B_0 axis and undetected. The acquisition sequence ($1331-180°_x-180°_y-180°_z$), like many multi-echo techniques, places emphasis upon the quality of the re-focusing 180° RF pulses. Like PRESS, MESA is principally used in the aquisition of ^1H spectra because the longer echo times (TE) can be exploited to distinguish between short T_2 "fat" resonances and the long T_2 found in the more interesting metabolites such as creatine, choline, N-actyl-aspartate and lactate.

● **Micro- milli-**
The prefix milli- is used to denote one thousandth of a particular unit. It is abbreviated to m. Similarly micro is used to denote a one millionth part and is abbreviated to μ. As such ms and μs become one thousandth and one millionth of a second respectively.

●**MOTSA**
This is an acronym of Multiple Offset Thin Slice Acquisition which is a technique used in MR angiography. Its main use is to improve the in-plane resolution without sacrificing coverage and reduce the "staircase" effect seen on sequences that use thicker slices.

● **Multi-slice imaging**
MRI pulse sequences must be repeated in order to build spatial encoding into signals.
The spatial encoding process is short, say 10.50 milli-seconds (ms), in comparison to the relaxation delays (TR) that are conventionally employed to manipulate image contrast (200-1500 ms). It is apparent that there is plenty of time when there is nothing to do except wait for relaxation to take place. If all radiofrequency (rf) pulses are made

slice-selective then this "dead time" can be usefully employed to acquire data from different slices in an interleaved fashion.
During the multi-slice imaging process the rf and gradient amplifiers are in use much more. To a close approximation an n-fold increase where n is the number of slices.
There is a relationship between the number of slices and the TR required. The slower the sequence runs (i.e. the longer TR) then the more slices can be squeezed into the available time. In some cases the user may be limited in the number of slices because the rf power deposition guidelines would be exceeded.

N

● **Nucleus**
The nucleus is the positively charged centre of an atom composed of a number of protons and neutrons (generically known as nucleons). Hydrogen, the simplest atom, contains only a single proton. The arrangements of these nucleons, both of which individually possess magnetic moments, determine the total nuclear magnetic moment of the nucleus.

● **Noise**
This comprises of electronic and acoustic forms. The random motions of electrons within conducting media constitute small, random electric currents. These currents give rise to spurious signals that can be detected by the sensitive MR receiver system. Electrolytes within the body, the copper within receiver coils and its associated cabling and connectors and electronic components all contribute to the overall noise level. The aim would always be limited by noise generated in the patient rather than the equipment.
The ratio of signal to noise (SNR) can be improved by the process of signal averaging. The signal, a coherent quantity, increases N-fold when the number of averages is N. Noise on the other hand is an incoherent process and accumulates as $\sqrt{N}$, where $\sqrt{}$ is the symbol for the square root. The net result upon the SNR is an improvement of $\sqrt{N}$; averaging four signals together, each with different noise, will improve SNR by a factor of 2. Similarly, averages of 9 or 16 will give SNR gains of 3 and 4 respectively. Under the simplest circumstances averaging will require an N-fold increase in scan time so there is a considerable penalty in terms of potential patient throughput.
Acoustic noise within the scanner results from the force generated with current is pulsed through the gradient coil system. The coil windings, although mechanically restrained, generate noise by moving against their restraint as the gradient current is increased. The mechanism is similar to the functioning of a loudspeaker coil. Since the magnitude of the force is related to the magnetic field strength and the current flowing in the gradient coils, a general rule would be that higher field systems are noisier than low field systems. Fast imaging techniques which require greater gradient usage, and therefore more switched current, also have a tendency to be noisier than their more sedate counterparts.

O

● **OVS – Outer Volume Suppression**
Spatial pre-saturation pulses are employed to attenuate the signals from unwanted regions. OVS is particularly useful in conjunction with ^1H spectroscopic localisation sequences that have shorter echo times (TE) where lipid/fat signals become problematic.

P

● **Paramagnetism**

The component atoms of a paramagnetic material possess permanent magnetic moments. The total moment of an individual atom has contributions from the unpaired orbiting electrons and from the central nucleus. Nuclear paramagnetism is several hundred times weaker than the electronic component. However the dominance of either will depend upon the particular atomic configuration. The atoms or ions of transition metals are typical examples of electronic paramagnetic substances.

An externally applied magnetic field will align, or polarise, these permanent magnetic moments and the bulk material will become magnetised. The extent of the magnetisation is inversely proportional to the absolute temperate (T); this is known as Curies' law. Electron paramagnetic resonance (EPR) relies upon the electronic contribution while nuclear magnetic resonance (NMR) employs the nuclear contribution to the overall paramagnetism of the material.

The presence of predominantly electronic paramagnetic ions, such as Gd^{3+} ions can substantially alter the relaxation properties of surrounding nuclear moments and this is the basis of the contrast agent. These ions are usually chelated to larger bio-acceptable molecules to reduce the toxicity although this does efficacy of the ions as relaxation agents.

● **Partial saturation**

When the time between radio-frequency (rf) pulses is less than or comparable to the longitudinal relaxation time (T_1) then a material is said to be partially saturated. Since there is insufficient time for full T_1 relaxation between rf pulses, the signal is certainly less than the equilibrium magnetisation (M_0) of the tissue. The varying extents of saturation amongst a variety of tissues with different T_1 are the basis for generating contrast in MR imaging.

In a more specific sense, the gradient echo sequence is often called the partial saturation sequence. This is the simplest of pulse sequences – a single rf pulse spaced at intervals TR. This sequence is also known as the field echo sequence. For fast imaging purposes a reduced rf pulse angle (less than 90°) is employed.

● **Phantom**

A test object to assess performance of the scanner. The phantom may contain water doped with paramagnetic Cu^{2+} or Mn^{2+} ions in order to control the relaxation times. As an alternative gels may be included since they may closer approximate to tissue where longitudinal relaxation times (T_1) are significantly longer than their transverse counterparts (T_2).

● **Phase**

The components of magnetisation constituting the MR signal can be imagined as the hand of a clock. It has a magnitude, the length of the hand, and a phase, how far it has rotated from the 12 o'clock position. In MRI we usually calculate an array of magnitudes only, display them on a two-dimensional grid and call them an image. Alternatively the phase of the signal may be computed, formatted to a grey scale and be presented as an image. Such practices have been useful in velocity phase encoding, where phase is linearly related to the velocity of blood for example, and field mapping where the phase is directly related to the magnetic field.

The phase of the magnetisation is taken with respect to some convenient orientation. In the above description, this was chosen to be 12 o'clock but this is purely arbitrary. It should also be noted that phase can only be calculated to within a single cycle. In the clock analogy, a hand pointing at 4 o'clock could be indicating am or pm of any day of the year. This dilemma can be resolved simply by observing or calculating the phase twice and displaying the difference between the two measurements.

The 90° and 180° nomenclature of radio-frequency (rf) pulses refer to phase angles. In this case it is the phase angle generated in the magnetisation during the time of the rf pulse. For the 90° pulse this would be from the preferred alignment along the magnetic field B_0 (z-axis) into the xy-plane. The 180° rf pulse can take magnetism from the +z to −z-axis, as in the inversion-recovery sequence, or alternatively in a spin echo simply move the magnetisation within the xy-plane.

● **Phase encoding**
The two-dimensional Fourier Transform (2DFT) imaging method has emerged as the dominant technique by which MR images are generated. Following slice selection magnetic field gradients are employed to localise the signal into a two-dimensional array of pixels. In the 2DFT scheme of imaging, one direction, which we can arbitrarily call the horizontal axis, is called the frequency encode axis. The vertical direction is called the phase encode axis. The frequency encoding can be envisaged as a number of phase encode steps collected in rapid succession during one pulse cycle.

Each pulse cycle under the 2DFT scheme employs a different phase encode gradient. Usually 128-256 different values would be employed to generate the image. A complete scan would then take 128-256 times the TR of the sequence.

For a static object the differences between phase and frequency directions are minimal. However for breathing or moving objects the fact that the phase encoding points are acquired every TR, rather than the faster rate of the frequency encoding, means this direction is the more sensitive with respect to movement.

● **Pixel**
Shorthand form for picture element. Each pixel within an MR image has a thickness, say 5mm, and this can lead to partial volume effects. Under these circumstances the term voxel (volume element) is perhaps more suitable.

● **Planar imaging**
MR signals are generated from the volume enclosed within, or in close proximity to, the receiver coil. By employing slice selective rf pulses, signals may be limited to planes within this volume. Additional field gradients are then employed to further spatially localise these signals in order to generate images. Planar imaging requires a decision as to the best imaging plane prior to the acquisition of the data. However, if sufficient numbers of narrow slices are produced, they can be employed to produce further oblique images.

As an alternative the signal from the volume may be manipulated without slice selective pulses. This is the volume scan which, once the data has been acquired, can be re-formatted to generate any arbitrarily oriented image plane.

● **Pre-amplifier**
The MR signal is very weak and can be easily swamped by noise. The pre-amplifier is an exceptionally low noise sub-system whose role is to magnify the basic MR signal (and noise) from the receiver coil without degrading it with additional noise. This initial amplification is the most critical and subsequent stages of the signal processing are more tolerant of lower quality components.

● **Precession**
The precession of nuclear magnets lies at the centre of the classical description of the nuclear magnetic resonance phenomenon. The static magnetic field (B_0) has a twisting effect upon the individual nuclear para-magnets. These magnets trace out a conical path around the direction of the field B_0 and this is known as precession. The nuclear precessional frequency is given by γB_0, and this is known as the Larmor frequency.

● **Pre-emphasis**
The close proximity of the gradient coil system to the structures of the magnet ensure that there is always a limited rise-time to the required changes in the gradient waveform. The changing current in the windings of the gradient coils induce currents within the bore of the magnet via magnetic interaction. This induced, or eddy current in the magnet stucture generates additional magnetic field gradients which are in opposition to those actually required. This non-ideal response can be reduced by pre-emphasising the initial sections of the input gradient drives.

● **PRESS – Point Resolved Surface Spectroscopy**
PRESS is a spin echo sequence that is used as a ^{1}H spectroscopic localisation technique. It employs three selective pulses, one in each of the three spatial axes x, y and z ($90°_x$-$180°_y$-$180°_z$), to leave signal from the required voxel to contribute to the final echo. It is particularly amenable to the acquisition of ^{1}H spectra where the comparatively long echo times (in the range 20-300ms or longer) can be integrated into the scan as an individual suppression of unwanted fat and lipid signals. The localisation pulses are preceded by a Chemical Shift Selective (CHESS) pulse in order to pre-saturate the large water resonance.

● **Pulse-collect**
The simplest of MR acquisition sequences involving a single RF pulse followed by the detection of the signal. The RF pulses are spaced at intervals of TR. If this interval exceeds 5 × T_1 then a 90° pulse should be employed to maximise signal-to-noise ratio (SNR). Reduced flip angles would be employed for faster TR and particularly when TR ~ T_1 or shorter. For *in-vivo* work a surface receiver coil is employed to reduce the area from which signal is detected. The pulse-collect sequence is often employed for ^{31}P and ^{13}C spectroscopic studies. The strong resonances from water and lipid preclude its usage in ^{1}H spectroscopy.

● **Pulse Sequence**
An MR pulse sequence consists of a series of radio-frequency (rf) and gradient pulses spaced by well defined time intervals. The rf pulses generate the MR signal. When applied simultaneously with a magnetic field gradient the rf pulses are slice selective, that is, MR signal is produced from only a slice of tissue. The signal can be further encoded with spatial information by the application of magnetic field gradients alone.

Pulse sequences repeat themselves with a periodicity of TR (seconds). Additional commonly occurring intervals are also defined; TE, the echo time and TI, the inversion time.

The MR pulse sequence may also include locking or synchronisation to physiological features such as the heart beat or respiratory motion.

Q

● **Q**
Q is the symbol for the quality factor of a tuned resonant circuit. A receiver coil, which is tuned to the nuclear Larmor frequency, with a high Q will resonate over a smaller range of frequencies than that of a low Q system. The signal-to-noise (SNR) of the detected MR signal is related to the Q of the coil; a high Q coil being most desirable in this respect. The proximity of a patient, or any conducting medium, to a tuned coil system will degrade its quality factor (and also SNR). The realistic measurement of Q will require "loading" of the coil with a suitable conducting material (or piece of anatomy).

● **Quadrature Coil**
A quadrature coil can be considered as two separate coils in close proximity to one another. Ideally they do not couple together so that the noise detected in each coil is uncorrelated. When these two noise signals are combined or averaged then the noise level is increased by $\sqrt{2}$.

The two coils are arranged to be perpendicular (90°) to one another. If the two signals are combined, taking into account this 90° in the receiver electronics, then overall signal is improved by 2. The net advantage of the quadrature coil is an improvement in signal to noise ratio (SNR).

The principal can be applied to transmitter coils when the advantage is more radio-frequency (rf) or B_1 field for the same power level from the rf amplifier. For the receiver coil there is a $\sqrt{2}$ improvement in SNR of the MR signal. If this improvement were sought by signal averaging alone then the scan time would be increased by a factor of 2.

● **Quench**
If the superconducting windings of a magnet were to become partially resistive then they immediately start to generate heat in the manner of an electric fire. The liquid helium bath, which maintains the low temperature for a superconducting state in the windings, starts to evaporate rapidly and this further accelerates the change of the magnet into a resistive state. This process is known as the quench of the magnet. There is a collapse of the magnet over several minutes and large quantities of helium gas are released from the magnet cryostat at great pressure. This would usually be vented to the atmosphere in order to reduce hazards.

R

● **Radio-frequency (rf)**
The relationship between frequency ν and magnetic field B is given by the Larmor equation ($\nu = \gamma B/2\pi$). For protons (^1H) at Tesla the frequency is 42.6MHz and, for the range of currently available magnets (say up to 12 Tesla for smaller bore systems), this puts the NMR frequency in the rf band of the electromagnetic spectrum The rf band is usually defined to lie in the frequency range of 10kHz to 100MHz. NMR is often referred to as an rf spectroscopy technique. The related technique of electron paramagnetic resonance (EPR) operates in the microwave portion of the electromagnetic spectrum.

The energy involved with each quantum or photon of rf radiation is low compared to typical molecular bond energies and this underlies the intrinsic safety aspects of MR when compared to X- and γ-rays towards the higher end of the electromagnetic spectrum.

The widespread use of rf in radio and television systems can lead to problems unless measures are taken to shield the MRI scanner from all interfering sources.

● **Receiver coil**
The detector of the MR signal is the receiver coil which would usually be designed to be fairly closely fitting to the anatomy in order to improve sensitivity. The receiver coil is tuned to the Larmor frequency which is defined by the field strength. The coil connects to a low noise pre-amplifier in order to boost the intrinsically low signals prior to meeting the outside world.

The receiver coil may physically be the same coil as the transmitter. In such cases additional electronics will be included in the transceiver system to switch between the high power transmit and the low power receive phases of its operation.

● **Relaxation**
The initial equilibrium polarisation of nuclear magnets or spins takes a finite time to evolve following positioning within the magnet. This time period is known as relaxation. Any non-equilibrium state of the nuclear magnetisation can only exist for a transitory period since relaxation processes are always working to maintain or restore the magnetisation along the B_0 field. These non-equilibrium states could be achieved by rapidly changing the magnitude or direction of B_0; in this case rapid means fast compared with the timescale or the relaxation processes. A more elegant approach is to apply rf pulses to realign the magnetisation away from its preferred orientation along B_0. The relaxation behaviour of nuclear spins, and in particular that of water (^1H), underpins the diversity of image contrast available in MRI.

Relaxation is described mathematically by the Bloch equations. The underlying message of these equations is that the relaxation of magnetisation should be considered as longitudinal and transverse to the magnetic field B_0. Longitudinal relaxation describes the re-growth of the M_z components of magnetisation along the field direction. Transverse relaxation describes the loss of any M_x and M_y components of magnetisation. Note that there is usually no distinction between the x and y components and the general transverse description is usually adequate.

Relaxation is promoted by the rotational and translation motions of the spins under investigation. For freely tumbling spins, as in liquids, the relaxation processes along and perpendicular to B_0 are identical. In more solid-like material the magnetic moments are not so free to move and transverse relaxation is faster than longitudinal re-alignment of magnetisation; the more solid, the greater the difference.

● **Repetition time (TR)**
The time between consecutive repetitions of a pulse sequence is labelled as TR. It is usual to say that if TR exceeds the five times the longitudinal relaxation time T_1 then full relaxation has occurred and the spin system has no "memory" of its previous history. Variations in the TR of a particular sequence can be employed to vary the T_1 contrast in the resultant image.

● **Resolution**
The smallest distance between distinct objects or features in an image. For a fixed field of view higher resolution requires a longer data acquisition period. The resolution of the acquired data is a function of the amplitude of the gradient pulses and their duration. The appearance of the processed image may be improved by interpolating the data to a finer matrix, however no additional detail results. Routine resolution in the plane of the image may be in the range 1-2mm and it might have a depth, or slice thickness, of perhaps 5mm.

● **Resonance**
A mechanical system such as a child's swing has a natural frequency at which it will oscillate if left to its own devices. If such an oscillatory system is drven by some periodic force then it will undergo forced oscillations. When the driver is at the natural frequency then resonance is said to have occurred; the amplitude of the oscillation builds up rapidly as energy is absorbed from the driver, in this case the exhausted parent. At other frequencies, slower and faster than the natural frequency, there is a flow of energy back and forth between oscillator and driver with no net gain by either system.
In MR the radio-frequency matches the quantum mechanical energy level splitting and transitions occur with a net energy absorption from the rf source. Since the energy levels are not infinitely sharp there is a narrow band of frequencies over which resonance between the MR spin system and rf source can be achieved. The energy absorption by the spin system is very small and should not be confused with the more generalised rf heating effects upon tissue.

S

● **Sampling**
The MR signal is a continuous voltage waveform that must be sampled or digitised into discrete steps for input into a computer prior to processing into an image. The sampling occurs at intervals in time during the evolution of the signal. During an MRI data acquisition the signal may typically be sampled every 10μsec. The voltage, which may now have been amplified to somewhere between −10 and +10 volts is digitised, for example, into one of 16384 discrete levels.
The artefacts associated with the failure to sample the signal correctly are commonly known. Aliasing occurs in the image when the signal is not sampled at sufficiently small intervals. If the voltage of the signal is too large then the input waveform is clipped or truncated; the appearance in the image is varied according to the extent of the overload.

● **Saturation**
If an equal number of spins are aligned with and against the magnetic field B_0, there is no net magnetisation in the tissue. This state is called saturation. Saturated tissue cannot contribute signal to a final image. This can be exploited to remove sources of artifact such as cardiac motion. Saturation can be achieved by repeatedly applying rf pulses at the Larmor frequency.

● **Selective excitation**
A radio-frequency pulse, by virtue of its limited duration, contains only a restricted range of frequencies, and as such can only excite a portion of the MR spectrum. Narrow excitation bandwidths are achieved with longer rf pulses. A pulse of duration tp seconds will have an approximate bandwidth of 1/tp Hertz; a 1ms (10^{-3}s.) pulse has a bandwidth in the region of 1 kHz (10^3Hz). By carefully tailoring the exact pulse shape and its carrier or centre frequency it is possible to selectively excite a given portion of the MR spectrum.

Selective excitation is employed in ^{1}H MRS to pre-saturate the strong water resonance prior to the acquisition of residual ^{1}H signals containing more specific molecular species (such as creatine, choline and N-acetyl aspartate). In such cases the Chemically Shift Selective (CHESS) rf pulses may be 40-50 ms in duration.

When combined with magnetic field gradients the selective frequency excitation becomes a spatially selective or slice selective pulse.

● **Shielding**
The interference caused by external rf sources such as hospital paging and computer systems can introduce artefacts and seriously degrade the signal-noise ratio of resultant MR images. The MR scanner is protected from its rf environment by Faraday shielding. ECG leads and other patient monitoring equipment that may breach the Faraday shield will have to be rf filtered to prevent interfering signals propagating through the wires.

The stray magnetic fields surrounding a whole body system can present a serious problem for cardiac pacemakers, visual display units and cathode ray tubes associated with monitoring equipment. There are NRPB guidelines concerning the general accessibility of regions where these stray fields may present some hazard. Magnetic flux lines cannot be attenuated in the sense of X-ray shielding but are simply re-directed through high permeability metals from which the magnet shield is manufactured.

● **Shimming**
The process of improving the quality of homogeneity of the static polarising field B_0 is known as shimming. The intrinsic inhomogeneity of a magnet in a particular hospital site can be improved at the time of installation with additional current carrying coils within the construction of the magnet itself. These shim coils may take currents of several amperes in order to generate additional corrective magnetic fields. As an alternative small pieces of ferromagnetic material can be accurately positioned within the bore of a magnet to produce a similar compensating and shimming effect.

Shimming may also be carried out on a per patient basis by observing the MR signal and improving its duration; the longer the signal in time, the smaller the range of frequencies it contains and the better the field over the region of interest. This may be achieved under computer control in many cases with an auto-shim procedure.

● **SI**
International standard of physical units and measures which supersedes the Metre-Kilogram-Second (MKS) and Centimetre-Gram-Second (CGS) systems.

● **Slice selection**
When an rf pulse is applied at the same time as a magnetic field gradient the frequency excitation can be expected to be heavily spatially dependent. If all pulses within a MR sequence are slice selective then during the necessary relaxation delays additional slices can be excited.

● **Specific Absorption Rate (SAR)**
Electromagnetic radiation can deposit energy by inducing small currents in the electrolytes of the body. The absorbed energy manifests itself principally in the form of heat. The specific absorption rate is defined as the energy deposited per second into a kilogram of tissue. It has the units of Watts per kilogram (W/kg). The energy absorption is limited to regions within the transmitter, or in close proximity to a surface transmitter, and as a result can be anatomically localised. The heat is generally dissipated by blood flow and as such, avascular structures such as the lens of the eye, are potentially at risk from rf

deposition. The National Radiological Protection Board (NRPB) limit the SAR to 0.4 W/kg in the whole body. For comparison, the threshold for production of cataracts is in the region of 100 W/kg.

● **Spectroscopy**

In the general sense spectroscopy is the separation of a signal into its component frequencies. The decomposition of white light into seven distinct colours is the common example. Spectroscopic techniques now exist throughout the electromagnetic spectrum from the lower radio-frequencies (NMR), electron paramagnetic resonance (EPR), infra-red, optical and ultra-violet and beyond. The methods are employed as probes to molecular and atomic structure.

In vivo magnetic resonance spectroscopy (MRS) is now commonly available on commercial high field systems (1.5T). High field is required since the separation of peaks is proportional to the field. The methods for the acquisition of spectra have converged on those employed in MRI with usage of magnetic field gradients to perform localisation either by slice selection and/or phase encoding. ^{1}H, ^{31}P, ^{13}C, ^{19}F and ^{23}Na have been studied to varying extents; ^{1}H MRS is now the most commonly investigated nucleus since the rf sub-systems of the scanner are identical to ^{1}H MRI.

● **Spin Warp**

Historically spin warp imaging arose as a method of image construction in competition with the back projection technique. It is now the predominate method employed to generate MR images due to its toleration of the artefactual effects of static field B_0 inhomogeneities. Spin warp imaging employs frequency and phase encoding to spatially resolve signals. Originally applied to planar imaging it has now been extended to volume imaging and the acquisition of MR spectroscopic data when multiple phase encoding directions are employed. The reconstruction of spin warp data is by a multi-dimensional Fourier Transform.

● **Spin echo**

The spin echo sequence consists of two rf pulses (90° and 180°) whose specific purpose is to re-focus the spin dephasing effects of the static field B_0 inhomogeneity and chemical shift. The 90° and 180° are separated by an interval of τ ms and the rephasing occurs τ ms after the 180° inversion pulse. The echo is formed TE after the initial 90° rf pulse, where TE is 2τ. This delay can be adjusted to generate T_2 contrast into the image. TE may typically lie in the range 10-80 msec although shorter and longer echo times may have specific applications.

● **Spin-lattice relaxation**

Spin-lattice or longitudinal relaxation describe the processes that cause the re-polarisation along the static magnet field B_0 Changes in the longitudinal magnetisation results from the redistribution or nuclear spins between their allowed quantum mechanical energy states. Quanta or discrete energy packs of rf radiation are either absorbed, as a spin makes a transition to a higher energy state, or emitted, when the reverse process occurs. The rf energy is considered to interchange between the spin system and a lattice, the local magnetic environment of the nuclear moments. The rate at which rf energy can flow between these two systems is dependent upon the availability of frequencies at the Larmor frequency. Molecular and sub-molecular translations and rotations are the source of the relevant rf frequencies and as such longitudinal relaxation measurements can be used to investigate the dynamical properties of systems. Molecular processes, and in particular the motion of water, are substantially altered by the presence of macromolecules such as proteins and cellular structures. In turn the measurable relaxation times T_1 will be observed to change by the proximity of such substrates.

● **Spin-spin relaxation**

Spin-spin or transverse relaxation describe the decay of the x and y components of the non-equilibrium magnetisation. The loss in these components arise from two processes; the re-alignment along the applied field (the z direction) and the irreversible dephasing of spins with respect to one another. The former of these two is the longitudinal or T_1

relaxation described beforehand. Dephasing occurs because individual spins that collectively contribute to the bulk magnetisation each experience a magnetic field that is dependent on their own local magnetic environment. Variations in fields can also occur because of practical imperfections in the B_0 field. Fortunately the spin echo can be employed to remove the experimental imperfections and produce the trie T_2 decay.

The transverse magnetisation is usually assumed to decay in an exponential manner and this description is included in the Bloch equations. However this is in no way fundamental and more complicated decays are often observed.

● Spiral scanning
This refers to a fast scanning technique where K-space is filled in a spiral fashion instead of the traditional linear pattern. The appearance of artefact can be considerably altered by changing the manner in which k-space is scanned.

● Steady-state
If a stream of rf pulses are applied at intervals less than the T_1 and T_2 of the sample then a steady state signal is produced.

The signal is present permanently, although it would not be possible to acquire data during the rf pulse itself since the receiver system is temporarily overloaded. A free induction decay (FID) follows each rf pulse while an echo signal appears prior to each pulse. The contrast obtained with steady state pulse sequences is apt to be limited. The contrast can be improved by sampling the "echo" part of the signal occurring before each pulse. The T_1 contrast is the same for FID and echo sections of the signal.

Steady state behaviour may be unwelcome, because of the low contrast attribute, and the use of "spoiling" gradients to dephase transverse components of magnetisation prior to each rf pulse tends to alleviate the problem.

● STEAM – Stimulated Echo Acquisition Mode
The STEAM sequence consists of three selective 90° pulses, one in each of the three spatial orientations ($90°_x$-$90°_y$-$90°_z$). During the interval after the second 90° pulse, the TM period, the required signal is orientated along the z-axis and so there is no loss in signal due to transverse relaxation. A stimulated echo is produced from the voxel of interest after the last 90° pulse and at a time equal to the spacing between $90°_x$ and $90°_y$. As with the multi-echo PRESS sequence, ^{1}H spectra can be acquired by preceding the STEAM localisation with a series of narrow band, CHESS water suppression pulses. Stimulated echoes are intrinsically half the intensity of their spin echo counterparts which would appear to be a considerable disadvantage. However voxel definition is superior, as a result of employing selective 90° rather than 180° pulses, and STEAM consistently provides shorter echo time sequences than its spin echo counterparts PRESS and MESA. STEAM has widespread use in the acquisition of ^{1}H spectra.

● Stimulated echo
The stimulated echo was described by Hahn at the same time as the spin echo, although it has a shorter history of usage in MRI and MRS. A stimulated echo is formed by any three rf pulses of arbitrary duration; it is most common to employ 90° pulses experimentally. The sequence can be written as 90° – TE/2 – 90° – TM – 90 – TE/2 such that the stimulated echo occurs (TE+TM) ms after the intial 90° pulse. (This description then matches the spin echo). During the period TM the required signal is "stored" along the z-direction, and as such the stimulated echo has a T_1 dependence related to the length of this period.

If the three rf pulses are slice selective then a volume is defined at the intersection of the three planes. Spectroscopic data can be obtained from this single voxel and as such the stimulated echo has widespread use in *in vivo* MRS.

● Superconductor
A material in which the electrical resistance is zero below a certain critical temperature. This temperature may lie in the region of 20K (20° above absolute zero) requiring the use of liquid Helium and liquid Nitrogen cryogens.

● **Suppression**

It is not uncommon in MR for there to be very strong signals in close proximity to more interesting but weaker areas. In MRI the intense lipid signals, exacerbated by the use of a surface coil, can dominate an image. In MRS the strong water resonance, representing 100 Molar ^{1}H, totally overwhelms the weaker spectroscopically interesting metabolite resonances. In both cases signal suppression techniques can be employed to reduce the amplitude of the offending signals.

Suppression techniques depend on distinct characteristic of the large signal. Spatial pre-saturation of a signal relies upon the differing location of the intense resonance and slice selective pulses can be employed to this end. The relaxation properties can be exploited, particularly with inversion recovery sequences, to null uninteresting signals. Short TI Inversion Recovery (STIR) and Fluid Attenuated Inversion Recovery (FLAIR) sequences are used to suppress lipid and CSF signals. The frequency of a particular resonance is determined principally by the field B_0 but also by the chemical shift interaction, and this can be exploited with selective excitation techniques such as CHESS (Chemical Shift Selective) or binomial (1331) pulses.

● **Surface coil**

A transmitter or receiver coil that does not envelope the body and as such has a very spatially dependent sensitivity profile. The high B_1-flux in close proximity to the coil can be exploited if MR is required from surface regions of the anatomy. A surface transmitter coil can produce intense rf pulses if required. As a receiver coil high quality images can be produced to a depth roughly equal to the radius of the surface coil.

T

● **TE, TI, TR**

American College of Radiology defined symbols for sequence timings. TE is the echo time, TI the inversion time and TR the repetition time of the sequence. TE is taken to be the time delay between the observation pulse, usually a 90° radio frequency (rf) pulse, and the data acquisition period of a sequence. As such TE is equally applicable to gradient-recalled and spin-echo sequences. An inversion recovery sequence, commonly realised as 180° – TI – 90°-180° in MRI, will actually have all three of these intervals associated with it.

● $T_1, T_2, T_2\star$

The time constants associated with longitudinal (T_1) and transverse (T_2) relaxation. These relaxation processes are usually assumed to be exponential in character and are given by the analytical solutions to the Bloch equations. In cases where this is not true then a sum of exponential relaxation processes may physically be a realistic model to allow characterisation of the relaxation behaviour.

Following a 90° rf pulse there is no component of magnetisation aligned along the applied field B_0; after a period of T_1 there will be 63% growth of the magnetisation along B_0 towards the equilibrium M_0. During T_2 transverse components of magnetisation decay by 63% from their initial value towards zero. Usually five times the relaxation time, either T_1 or T_2, is taken to be the time necessary for the respective components of nuclear magnetisation to fully relax.

$T_2\star$ is employed to denote the actual observed decay in transverse relaxation. The distinction is required since $T_2\star$ depends upon the experimental conditions under which the signal is observed to be decaying. In the simplest case, in the absence of imaging field gradients following a single rf pulse for example, this means that the field inhomogeneity (δB_0) can also contribute to the decay of the MR signal.

● **Tesla**

Named after Nikola Tesla (1870-1943), the Tesla is the SI unit of magnetic flux density and is given the symbol T. Commercial MR scanners usually operate in the range 0.2-2.0T. One Tesla equates to 10000 (10^+) Gauss, the equivalent CGS unit.

● **TMR – Topical Magnetic Resonance**
Topical Magnetic Resonance was an early spectroscopic localisation technique that relied upon the very selective shimming to a small region in space. The higher order spatial harmonics of the magnetic field B_0 were designed to limit the size of the homogeneous volume from which high quality spectra can be obtained. A specially designed magnet is required for this technique. Signals outside and on the periphery of this volume are inhomogeneously broadened and are either absent from the signal or can be removed by post-processing. The homogeneous volume from which the signal is derived is not particularly well-defined and there is very little control over its position and dimensions. Re-alignment of the patient is required in order to achieve this level of control.

● **Transmitter coil**
A coil system capable of handling high rf current. The current as it flows around the coil, generates a time dependent or rf magnetic field; this is generally referred to as B_1 to compare with the static polarising field B_0. The current in the transmitter coil is switched on and off, or pulsed, under computer control in order to generate the required rf pulse sequences.
A body sized transmitter coil is widely applicable to all parts of the anatomy. However, by virtue of its size, high power is required in order to generate the required 90° and 180° rf pulses. Furthermore all of the body within the coil is irradiated with subsequent increase in rf absorption (SAR). Smaller head coils are also available in order to reduce the power requirements and reduce SAR.

● **Transverse magnetisation (M_{XY})**
These are the non-equilibrium components of the magnetisation that exist perpendicular to the applied fields B_0 (which defines the z axis). Transverse magnetisation is usually generated as a result of a 90° rf pulse, the 90° being the angle between z and the transverse xy-plane.
The precession of the transverse magnetisation at the Larmor frequency induces a voltage in the receiver coil and this constitutes the basic MR signal. The signal will decay in a time $T_2^\star$ and experimental conditions such as the quality of the magnetic field and the size of the region from which the signal is derived.

● **Transverse relaxation**
The equilibrium magnetisation is aligned along the z-axis, defined by the static magnetic field B_0 and there are no components in the transverse or xy-plane. Following a rf pulse any transverse magnetisation must decay to zero and this occurs at the molecular level by transverse relaxation mechanisms.

● **Tuning**
The adjustment of the frequency to a specific value where resonance can occur is known as tuning. The concept is familiar when selecting a specific ratio station. In MR terms the rf system must be matched to the Larmor frequency (v_0) defined by the field B_0 ($v_0 = \gamma B_0/2\pi$). Individual coils within the MR system, be they high powered transmitter coils or receiver coils, must also be tuned to the Larmor frequency for optimum performance.

V

● **Velocity encoding**
Phase Contrast Angiography will display both arterial and venal flow in the same slice unless velocity encoding is utilized. By setting the encoding velocity (Venal flow e.g. 15cm/sec, venous flow can be displayed. A Venc of 500cm/sec is necessary to demonstrate arterial flow.

● **Voxel**
Shorthand form for the volume element of an image. Voxel emphasises that the smallest image element not only has an inplane dimension also has a thickness or depth.

● **Volume Imaging**
In the absence of any magnetic field gradients all parts of the body within the transmitter coil are excited by an rf pulse. If the receiver coil surrounds a large volume of this excited region then the signal can be manipulated for volumetric imaging.
Volume imaging can be achieved with frequency encoding and two phase encode axes – a three dimensional Fourier transform (3D-FT) technique. A volume scan will take n times longer than its planar equivalent, where n is the number of points required in the third dimension. Unless n is large then a multi-slice dataset may be competitive in terms of coverage of the required anatomy.
Volume scanning is a most efficient way of acquiring data from an extended volumetric region. However, the use of the second phase encoding axis can make scan times rather long and, as a result, volume scanning tends to go hand in hand with fast imaging techniques. Such techniques may include reduced angle rf pulses and echo planar imaging methods. The resultant image data has voxels which are more isotropic (equal resolution in each of the three spatial directions) than a set of multi-slice images. In multi-slice imaging the in-plane resolution is usually much better than the slice thickness. Planes of many orientations can be derived from a single volume scan, perhaps on a separate workstation.

● **VSE – Volume Selective Excitation**
VSE is a single shot localisation technique based upon a composite selective procedure ($45°_x$-$90°45°_x$) where both the 45° pulses are slice selective (x) and the 90° is broadband. The required "in-slice" material is inverted longitudinally while the unwanted magnetisation is left in the transverse plane. Care must be taken to avoid the generation of stimulated echoes. Three orthogonal composite slice selection pulscs, a total of nine pulses in all, are required to define a single voxel. VSE requires high rf power if the gradient is *not* switched during the broadband 90° pulse. VSE has been applied to the acquisition of ^{13}C and ^{31}P spectra. A variant called SPARS (SPAtially Resolved Spectroscopy) alleviated some of these limitations by switching the gradient pulses during the RF sequence.

X, Y, Z

● **x, y, z**
These refer to the three principal axes in a Cartesian co-ordinate system, that is the usual rectangular system that can be applied to rooms, buildings and the like. X, y and z are said to be in the laboratory frame of reference if they are attached to the system hardware associated with the MR scanner. Convention has it that the applied magnetic field defines the z-axis of the co-ordinate system. Since the majority of systems today are based upon the superconducting solenoid magnet this means that z runs from head to foot in the patient. The x and y axes are not only perpendicular to z but also at right angles with respect to each other.

● **x′, y′, z′**
These also refer to a Cartesian system of co-ordinates but the inclusion of the superscript prime indicates that these axes refer to a rotating frame of reference. The choice of the "rotation" is entirely arbitrary but is selected to simplify the description of the movements of nuclear magnetisation. This is true for the visualisation in the mind and also the underlying mathematics. In MR the rotating frame is usually taken to be attached to the precession of a particular group of nuclei in the magnetic field. As such the z and z′ axes are one and the same and the x, y and x′, y′ axes are simply rotating with respect to one another. The literature is apt to be rather loose about the co-ordinate system or frame of reference in which nuclei or magnetisation are being discussed.

● **Zero Alternate phase (ZAP)**
The ZAP sequence is a modification of the FISP sequence. A stream of evenly spaced rf pulses are used which result in the accumulated gradient phase of O on alternate intervals instead of all intervals (as in FISP). The ZAP sequence produces a true FISP-like signal without the magnetic field inhomogeneity banding artifacts of FISP.

● **Zeugmatography**
A term coined from Greek roots to mean MRI. Positively the last word in Magnetic Resonance Imaging.

NOTES

NOTES